OUT OF THE DARKNESS

SURVIVING MIGRAINES

AND HEADACHES

JENNIFFER RABE

ISBN-13: 978-1475208962
ISBN-10: 1475208960

Dedicated to the millions of migraine and headache sufferers;

You are not alone in your struggles.

Special thanks to my wonderful doctors: Dr. R. Vollbract and

Dr. K. Dean for helping me to deal for all these years.

To my family and close friends; thank you for always being
supportive.

CONTENTS

LIVING WITH MIGRAINES

I would like to start by telling you a little about myself and my struggles with migraine headaches.

I am thirty-four years old and I have had migraine headaches for the past twenty years. When I was fifteen I suffered from a severe head injury. I never had a headache before my injury. Since then I have daily headaches and chronic migraines.

I have to say my choices the night of my injury were definitely bad ones. I could say I was just being a teenager doing teenage things but the more accurate way to summarize it is I was just being stupid.

At the time, I was living in an apartment complex. I was supposed to have been home for the night. My mom was not home and I thought I could get away with staying out a little later than I was supposed to. Approximately ten to fifteen teens from the neighborhood were hanging out at the basketball/tennis courts. Some were playing basketball, some were hanging out with their friends; laughing and having a good time, and some were drawing obscene chalk drawings on the ground. Two older guys were at the tennis net and thought it would be funny for someone to sit on the tennis net and they would fling them in the air. The way this worked is someone would sit on the tennis net; there was a guy on both sides of that person. They would each push down and then pull the net back up which would catapult the person sitting on the net. I was watching this and it looked really fun. The people that were flung would go approximately one to two feet in the air and land on their feet. So I did it. The first time I did it I did not land on my feet; I landed on my butt. It was a rush and I wanted to do it again. My best friend begged me not to but I didn't listen to her. The second time I did it, I was flung *much* higher in the air. There were people at different parts of the neighborhood who said the saw me go higher than the fence around the tennis net; almost parallel to the two-story apartment building next to the courts. I flipped through the air landing on my head on the cement tennis court. I hit my head/face in three places. My eye was swollen shut; I had a huge knot behind my ear and one on the back of my head. According to the paramedics and Doctors I passed out while in the air. Apparently my subconscious saw what was coming and passed out. I was told passing out prior to impact is what saved my life.

I don't remember a lot from that day. I remember asking repeatedly if my friend could come to the hospital with me and that my first name was not spelled right on my hospital armband. Some events I still do not remember.

From that day on I have suffered from daily headaches and chronic migraines. Logically, you would think I have a head or neck injury or pinched nerve causing my migraines. I had a concussion that night of course, however after twenty years, more tests than I can count and numerous doctors; I apparently have what is referred to as "classic" migraines. All my tests have come back "negative" which means there is nothing abnormal going on up there (although I know some people who wouldn't agree). I am told my migraines are hereditary. I do not know of anyone in my family who suffers from migraines. Some sinus headaches from time to time but no one in my family has headaches like I do. So what could that possibly mean "hereditary"? I am sure a lot of you can relate in one way or another. It is hard to find a doctor that is able to help. I have seen a lot of different neurologists over the past twenty years. At the time, most of them seemed like "pushers" to me. Every time I went to a neurologist my medication dosage was increased and more were added. By the time I was seventeen the top of my dresser was seventy-five percent covered in prescriptions. I was heavily medicated. I remember lying in my bed, my room pitches black and I couldn't move. My pillow felt as though I were laying on a cinder block. If I even moved my eyes I would vomit. I quickly got tired of the doctors and of all the medications. I just wanted a doctor who would find out *why* I was getting migraines and fix it, not just prescribes a lot medication and hope one would do the trick. I had almost given up on neurologists until my primary doctor told me about the neurologist I am currently seeing. She said there were studies and research done on Botox for migraines and I most likely would be a good candidate. My current neurologist has helped me more than any other and I have been with him nearly five years now. There are good neurologists out there. Guess it's like trying to find the perfect partner for you; you have to weed through some bad ones to find the perfect one for you and what may be your perfect one is not always someone else's.

As I mentioned, over the years, I have been on a *substantial* amount of medications. A lot are known to help headache or migraines but were specifically made for other reasons such as blood-pressure or antidepressants. The most commonly used medications for migraines are *triptans*. The best thing I have heard about those specific medications is that they do not cause drowsiness making it perfect for when you need to be alert such as at work.

I am personally unable to take any type of medication in the triptan family. I can have a severe migraine and when I take any type of triptan my migraine intensifies excessively. It is as if I was hit by a Mack truck and it is parked on my head. However triptans are successful for a lot people. There will always be pros and cons with any medication and some people are more sensitive than others.

I went through numerous different medications and corticosteroid injections finding little relief before I was found to be a good candidate for Botox (onabotulinum toxin type A) which has been shown to improve migraine headaches. I have been receiving the Botox injections for several years now. I have found Botox helpful compared to before I began treatment. As with all medications there are side effects and everyone is different. My most noticeable side effect for Botox is that my hair went from straight hair to curly at and near the injection sites. I rarely had a bad hair day until about a year after I began Botox and now my hair gets frizzy. As with the cosmetic Botox, the medicinal Botox also tightens the skin. I receive a lot of injections most of which in the base of my scull, some in my trapezoids, near my shoulder blades, at my hairline and several spots on my face (near my eyes, and temples). I basically receive the injections where I experience my pain.

 In the early part of 2011 my migraines were getting substantially worse and I was hospitalized for three days under the orders of my neurologist. I was admitted so they could administer DHE (dihydroergotamine) intravenously (via IV). From what I have been told and what I have found while researching, DHE is a medication that has helped with severe migraines since 1943. Unfortunately, this is another medication I seem to have a reaction to. During my 2011 hospital stay I was given DHE. Within the first thirty seconds of the drug being injected into my IV I had a very bad reaction. I was first given Reglan to coat my stomach and aid in nausea and was then given the DHE slowly through my IV. The nurse had given me maybe half of the injection when I reacted. I began to experience an intense pressure in my head/brain, different and much more severe than any I had experience before. I tried to be still and just hoped it would pass. I thought maybe it is like some other injections that hurt or are uncomfortable while being administered then subside. Unfortunately, the pressure got much worse. I found that I couldn't be still. The nurse continued to administer the DHE and the pressure grew stronger and unbearable. The nurse stopped and call for the doctor. It felt as though my head was going to explode and I was beyond uncomfortable. For the remainder of my three day stay I was not given DHE again. I have read more about this medication since my hospital visit and studies do show it effective for Status Migraines (*Status Migraines* are headaches that do not go away with the traditional treatments) I just added this to the growing list of what doesn't work for me.

When I was released from the hospital I felt as though I was in a drug-induced fog or a *virtual* reality. It took over a week until that drugged feeling went away. I have to tell you, that "drugged" feeling is pretty scary especially when it last for days. With that in mind along with the fact that nothing I had been doing appeared to be working and the list of medications I was taking just kept getting longer; I decided to wean off of all my medications (under doctors supervision of course). I don't know if I was on too many medications and maybe they began working against each other. I have *heard* that you should not take

11

more than five active medications or supplements at any one time. I believe it has something to do with the effectiveness and absorption of the medication in your body.

It took some time to get completely weaned off all the medications. Some I had really awful withdrawal and others weren't that hard at all. I only weaned off one medication at a time so I could observe what I was feeling and how long I was having the withdrawal. Once I was completely weaned off of one, I could determine if my headaches/migraines were better or worse.

After a couple months, everything was completely out of my system. I'd had daily pain from either a bad headache to a severe migraine as well as daily nausea for as long as I can remember. The only thing that changed was the severity of the two. All of a sudden, I had a day without pain and nausea. I couldn't believe it. The next day was the same. I was shocked but didn't want to think too much about it for fear I would jinx it and they would come back. Then, on the second virtually pain-free evening something odd happened. I began to see brightness in the center of my vision as if I had just stared into the sun and looked away. Within a half hour I had lost my peripheral vision. Of course this freaked me out. I wondered, "*Is this some new symptom? Am I about to get slammed with an excruciating migraine? Great, what now?*"

It did past after about half hour and I was fine for the rest of the night. The next morning, I didn't have a severe migraine. I did however have pressure behind my eyes and the top of my head and in my right temple. I called my neurologist and I was told it sounds like another symptom to my headaches/migraines. I recently had an MRI and once again it came back "negative". On the MRI they also checked to make sure I didn't have an aneurism. Let's face it, when our headaches or even the symptoms change from what we are used to experiencing the first thing we all do is panic and worry it could be an aneurism or something terrible, I know I do. There usually isn't any warning with aneurisms. And from what I am told most of time you do not experience headaches with tumors.

Since then, I have more days with less severe headaches. I still have them, both headaches and migraines. It may have been hormones that caused the change. At this point I am unsure. I do get pressure especially in the back of my head and neck area. At times they are still intense, but nothing like what I have experienced almost daily for the past twenty years. I am worried they may come back as intense as before. However, I am glad to have some type of life. It is depressing and difficult to have to be cautious and aware of every little thing in fear it will cause or worsen your migraine. Light and smells are triggers for me. It is somewhat exciting to be able to do things you had to mainly avoid such as have your blinds open to allow the light to come in. I love nature and beautiful sunny days and yet at times I have to avoid the light. Even in the overcast it would still affect me. It's nice to be able to come *Out of the Darkness.*

The more I research, the more I hear about people such as myself who have migraine or severe headaches that also do not find relief from the typical migraine treatments. It is good to know I am not alone in this daily struggle and at the same time it's terrible to know that there are so many people who experience what I do.

That is why I decided to write this. I want to put my experience along with what I have learned in one place for everyone who wants or needs the information. Perhaps someone will find the answers they seek or another idea to try. I wish everyone relief from their pain.

Tension Headaches

Tension headache is a common type of headache and experienced by most people at one point or another in a life time. Generally over-the-counter (OTC) medications are helpful in alleviating this type of headache pain.

Although tension headaches are common, their symptoms and causes are more complicated than we realize. Just because it is called a "Tension" headache does not necessarily mean it is caused by tension.

Everywhere you look for information regarding tension headaches you will see that there are two-types of headaches; Episodic and Chronic.

An episodic headache occurs at random. This type is often caused by stress, anxiety and fatigue.

When you experience the episodic tension headache you could experience a constant, non-throbbing dull ache, soreness in the temples, a tight band-like feeling around your head, pressure, what feels like pulling and a tightness of the head or neck muscles. This tightness in the neck and head could also feel like your head or neck is restrained and difficult to move with very few positions of relief.

If you unconsciously tense up your head and neck muscles in response to stress you may find that your scalp is tender or your neck and shoulder muscles are especially tight.

This type of headache usually appears in the temples, forehead, back of head and/or neck.

If you can find relief with OTC medication then they are probably episodic headaches. These can occur several times in a month, they are easily maintained with OTC medications, mild exercise and a good night's sleep.

The second type is a chronic tension headache. Chronic tension headaches may also be caused by stress or fatigue, but generally they are caused from physical problems such as injuries; psychological issues and depression.

This type of headache can affect both men and women but women seem to be more susceptible. The difference between episodic headaches and chronic headaches is the frequency and severity of the symptoms. The symptoms for chronic headaches are similar to that of the episodic headaches.

The common physical symptoms of a chronic tension headache are muscle constriction between your head and neck which can last for days. Some experience tightness or pressure around your neck and the base of the scull. You may experience soreness, a tightening band of pressure around your head as if your head is in a vice. As well as a "pulling" sensation in your neck and/or head.

For most people with this type of headache the pain is continuous, very annoying but not a throbbing pain. It is mainly pressure. It generally occurs in your forehead, temples, the back of your head and neck.

This could also be a symptom of anxiety and depression. Most people do not realize they are depressed nor have anxiety. Either way, depression and anxiety are a symptom or result of chronic tension headaches. You may feel fine and not depressed or anxious at all however there could be something happening in your life causing depression or anxiety. Depression doesn't have to be a state of sadness or lack of emotional control. You don't have to have chest pains for example to have anxiety. Try to figure out if something is bothering you such as a loss of some sort or stress because you cannot pay your bills and your financial situation has been going on for some time without relief. That alone could cause some form of depression as well as anxiety. Also see your physician and discuss what is going on in your life. Most people hold in emotions of all sorts and that is not good for your emotional wellbeing and at some point can affect your physical wellbeing.

If you have a change in your sleep patterns such as not enough sleep or sleeping too much this could also cause chronic headaches. This is also a symptom of anxiety and depression. Do you have Insomnia or difficulty falling asleep? Do you wake up earlier then you want to? All of this can be attributed to headache, anxiety and/or depression.

Think back and ask yourself if you experience any of the following:

Shortness of breath

Nausea

Weight loss

Weight gain

Ongoing fatigue

Decreased sex drive

Dizziness

Unexpected crying

Being upset over something that generally would not upset you

Change in your menstruation (such as heavier, lighter, late or lack of).

All of the above listed symptoms could be related to depression or anxiety and attribute to chronic headaches. If you experience any of those symptoms talk to your physician. Make sure he or she knows of these changes this way you can be properly diagnosed. Medication may be required. With all medications, make sure your doctor AND pharmacist are aware of everything you are taking so there aren't any drug interactions. I always use the same pharmacy so that nothing gets missed. I recommend talking to your pharmacist, having a second person reviewing your medications is always a good idea. A pharmacist works strictly with medications day in and day out. So they are the perfect source for questions regarding medications, side effects and interactions. Supplements (herbs, vitamins, minerals etc.) should always be addressed as well. They could have a reaction with a chemical medication. Better safe than sorry.

There are also physical causes for tension headaches such as poor posture, bad lighting or having you head/neck in an unnatural position for an extended length of time. People who work in an office and work on computers could easily experience headaches due to the environment and length of time they are working. Eye strain, loud noises and bright lighting are also key factors.

All these physical problems can be corrected in some form. Each person is different in what could cause or correct any type of headache.

I have had numerous people tell me that a Chiropractor was helpful for them. I have tried several Chiropractors during various stages of my migraines and although I feel better right after the first initial visit (aside from soreness) I feel worse later that day and the next few days. Chiropractic usually doesn't work for me. Message therapy is another option. I would recommend a sports therapist. Your doctor could refer you and most insurance cover this. You can also find a list of all doctors and therapists on your insurance companies' website.

With all headaches, there are two things we all work towards; prevention of future headaches and getting rid the current headache. I have found that people who don't experience severe headaches do not understand the affects they have on our lives.

I have found myself thinking on more than one occasion "I wish they would have *just one* migraine. I bet they'd understand then." Not that I wish this on anyone, I just wish for the understanding. I have had to leave work early or not been able to go in at all. I have not been able to do things with my son. If it is too hot or humid outside, I cannot be out for any length of time. The migraine will get so intense I can't function. My body is exhausted when I come home from work, basically from fighting the headache all day. When I get home I let my defenses down and exhaustion sets in. There is a constant nausea. It is extremely difficult to live with them in all aspects of life. And when the medications and treatments don't work, it makes you want to give up. Unfortunately, that is not an option.

In some instances, tension headaches go away when you slow down and relax; take some deep breaths. Do something that allows you to relax, stretching exercises or even a warm bath.

Migraine Headaches

When you have a migraine headache you know it. And for that matter so do the people around you. These vicious headaches can disrupt every facet of your life. There are millions of people in the world who suffer from migraines. I don't want to give a specific or even an estimated number because the statistics found do not include people who do not report it or seek medical assistance and information changes faster than we realize. Say you are reading this book a year after I wrote it; the statistics will undoubtedly have changed.

Women experience migraines more than men do. This is due to hormonal changes that take place in women, whether it is during menstruation or the hormonal changes throughout our lifetime. Most migraine sufferers tend to be certain types of people such as perfectionists, high strung, analytical and critical. The word migraine is from the Greek word *hemicranias" meaning "half of the head"*.

Until recently, most clinicians believed migraines to be a vascular condition, caused by the blood vessels in your head dilating. It has recently been found that migraine is much more complex. It is now though that there are multiple mechanisms that contribute to the onset of migraine a while before any pain is felt.

The multi-mechanism approach suggests that the headache pain results from a chain of both vascular and neurological events. It is said that migraine pain is caused not only by vasodilatation (the widening of blood vessels) but begins with inflammation leading to norciception (pain receptors) and central and peripheral sensitivity.

This new understanding may also explain why many migraine sufferers may experience a variety of uncommon symptoms, such as face and sinus pain in addition to the common pain and symptoms.

There are many factors that can trigger a migraine, such as changes to sleep or waking cycle, missing or delayed meals, some medications; daily or near-daily use of medications designed for migraine relief; bright lights, sunlight, fluorescent lighting, TV and movie viewing; certain foods, excessive noise, odors and physical activities. Stress and/or depression are important factors that can help with diagnoses and treatment of migraine headaches. Keeping a headache diary can be very effective for yourself as well as your doctor. You can become aware of what your triggers are and make a conscious effort to avoid them.

The two most common types of migraines are migraine with aura and migraine without aura. Migraine with aura is referred to as "classic" migraine whereas migraine without aura is referred to as "common" migraine.

Most migraine sufferers experience two to four headaches per month. Some people get them every day while others may get them one or two times a year. Most migraines last at least four hours however very severe ones can last a week or longer. You can get a headache at any time of the day or night. You could wake with a migraine but rarely be awaken from sleep due to a migraine.

A migraine often starts with a dull ache and then develops into a constant throbbing and pulsating pain. This pain can become intense very quickly. You could begin feeling the pain at the temples as well as the front or back of one side of the head. The pain is usually accompanied by nausea and/or vomiting, and sensitivity to light and/or sound.

While some migraine sufferers do experience visual problems during the headache, you could be one who has aura as a warning sign prior to the pain. For me, I see bright light spots as well as black spots floating in my vision prior to the onset. It comes and goes and then the migraine hits me.

It usually takes anywhere from twenty to thirty minutes from when the spots appear to when the migraine starts. Aura is visual disturbances. You could see wavy or jagged lines, dots or flashing lights. Some people get tunnel vision or blind spots in one or both eyes. You could experience vision or hearing hallucinations and smells or odors and tastes could bother you.

Some people experience numbness or a tingling "pins and needles" feeling. There could also be a loss in concentration, difficulty finding the word(s) you are trying to say or even speaking clearly. These symptoms should fade once the headache has started. Once the migraine attack is full-blown, many people will become sensitive to anything that touches their head as well as some movements.

Other types of migraines are rarer such as hemiplegic migraine, retinal migraine, basilar artery migraine and abdominal migraine.

With hemiplegic migraine, you often experience temporary motor paralysis and sensory disturbances on one side of your body followed by the headache within an hour. You may also have the "pins and needles" feeling or numbness. These symptoms usually subside once the headache has started.

With retinal migraine you will either temporarily, partially or completely lose your vision in one eye followed by a dull ache behind that eye that could spread to the rest of your head.

A basilar type migraine is a migraine with aura. The aura symptoms come from both sides of the brain or the brainstem. It is most common in young adults. The symptoms for this type of headache include dizziness, double or blurred vision, loss of balance, confusion, slurred speech, hearing changes and tingling on both sides of the body. During an attack, some people can lose consciousness or pass out. The aura usually last less than an hour. Sometimes people with these symptoms are thought to be intoxicated. The headache that follows these symptoms is usually described as a typical migraine.

Ophthalmoplegic migraines are severe and rare. The pain usually surrounds the eyeball and can last for a few days to a few months. You could also experience paralysis in the muscles surrounding your eye. If you continue to get this type of migraine, see a doctor; you may have pressure on the nerve behind the eye.

Migraine can also be associated with serious results such as aura lasting longer than a week with or without stroke and migraine-triggered seizures. If you or someone you know experiences one of these rarer migraine headache types it is important to see a specialist to get diagnosed and treated. People with these types of headaches and symptoms should also avoid the triptan family of medications.

There are a lot of ways to treat and prevent migraines. Sometimes the treatments are not as effective as we would like them to be but with a large number of people they are quite effective.

It is important to pay attention to the types of foods you eat as some may be a trigger. It is also important to have normal eating and sleeping habits. Try going to bed and waking up the same time every day. I realize this is not always possible, but this type of routine could be quite helpful. Also a regular exercise routine (nothing exerting), avoiding nicotine and alcohol may be helpful in managing migraines and headaches. There are also therapies such as acupuncture, biofeedback and physical therapy that may be helpful.

Coexisting Migraine and Tension Headaches

Some people describe having both daily chronic tension headache and a recurring migraine headache. This headache combination was previously known as mixed headaches syndrome but is now known as coexisting migraine and tension headaches. Other terms used include: transformation migraine, chronic migraine and chronic daily headaches. People who experience these types of headaches are more prone to experience rebound headaches from overuse of analgesics, ergot and triptan medications.

Most people who experience these types of headaches have a previous history of periodic migraine that began around adolescence to their twenties. The daily, milder headache tends to form later in life. Some people with coexisting migraine and tension headaches have a history of daily headaches which are at times more severe and may have been accompanied by migraine symptoms such as nausea and/or vomiting and sensitivity to light or sound. Some people may have had a long history of migraines where the severity will decrease but they still have one on a daily basis. It may be hard to tell the difference between the two types of headaches. One way to tell if you do experience a coexisting migraine and tension headache is by asking yourself how many headaches do you experience, this is another way the headache diary comes into play.

You may be able to tell by the symptoms experienced however many of the symptoms may be vague. The hard or severe type may be one-sided and associated with nausea, vomiting and sensitivity to light and/or sound (migraine like) whereas the daily headache may be on both sides, mild to moderate in severity and feel like a vise around your head (tension like). Misdiagnosis happens a lot with these types of headaches and the treatment given is more likely to treat one of these types instead of both.

Due to the chronic nature of these types of headaches people tend to overuse OTC medications as well as some "rescue" type medications. They take them on a daily or near daily basis. Some will use large amounts of caffeine in beverages and analgesic. The most commonly overused are narcotic pain relievers such as Vicodin, Hydrocodeine and butalbital containing prescriptions such as Fioricet. Excedrin is an OTC analgesic pain reliever that contains caffeine. You can even over use the ergotamine or triptan family of medications. As my doctor explained you should not use any rescue pain relieving medication more than ten to fifteen days per month. When you stop taking overused medications you will most likely experience withdrawal headaches for several days then your headaches should feel somewhat better.

Many people who experience coexisting migraine and tension headaches have a coexisting medical issue like hypertension or a psychiatric disease like depression. There are anti-depressants that are useful in treating depression that are also helpful with headaches and migraines because of their analgesic properties. You may also be prescribed anti-epileptic drugs such as Topimax (topiramate) which has been found helpful when used in combination therapies.

People who do not respond to treatment are sometimes sent for non-medication treatments such as biofeedback or physical therapy. You should avoid all medications that may lead to dependency when dealing with this type of headaches.

CLUSTER HEADACHES

Cluster headaches are rare; only a small percentage of the population experience cluster headaches. It is said that men experience cluster headaches more than women do. Cluster headaches are one of the most painful types of headache. They are said to be excruciating and even more debilitating than a migraine. Cluster headaches were at one time considered a type of migraine because it is a vascular headache.

The symptoms of a cluster headache are typical. The pain arrives with little or no symptoms. You generally do not experience aura or visual disturbances or nausea with these types of headaches. The head pain is almost always on one side and stays in the same area during the attack. The pain can begin on the opposite side when a new headache begins. The pain is usually intense and severe; described as sharp like a nail or knife stabbing or piercing around the eye or centered over one eye, to the temple, forehead and cheek. It may cause one of the eyelids to become swollen or droop. It can also be accompanies by a tearing or bloodshot eye. The nostrils on the affected side may become congested and become runny. At times people may experience excessive sweating or the face on the affected side may become flush. It can spread to a larger area making it difficult to diagnose.

There are several things that can trigger a cluster headache: alcohol, becoming over-heated, exercise and strong odors such as paint fumes, gas, perfume, bleach, chemicals and smoke such as cigar smoke. Try to avoid these types of triggers especially during an attack.

During a cluster headache the pain is usually experienced at approximately the same time every day. The headache usually starts at night waking you from sleep an hour or two after you have fallen asleep. The pain will generally reach its intensity within five to ten minutes and will stay that intense for approximately thirty minutes to an hour. The length of time depends on the person. It could last for fifteen minutes or for several hours. Unfortunately the headache could resurface during the day.

For people with bouts of cluster headaches, the head pain can last for four days to two weeks usually during the spring and/or autumn. After that it could disappear for a few months or years. This type of cluster headache is an episodic cluster headache.

Cluster headaches are often associated with allergies. A small percentage of cluster headache sufferers experience chronic cluster headaches that occur all year long. People with cluster headaches usually have a difficult time keeping still during an attack and often try to alleviate the pain by walking around or pacing, sometimes even banging their head against the wall until the pain subsides.

Unlike migraine headaches, cluster headaches are not thought to be hereditary. Sufferers usually do have a history of chronic smoking and frequently drink alcohol which can trigger a cluster headache. The histamine levels increase during a cluster headache. It has not yet been proven but antihistamines which dilate or expand your blood vessels may be helpful.

Hormonal Headaches

Both men and women's headaches are prompted by hormones, generally only women suffer from hormone headaches. You would not feel pain if it weren't for hormones. Hormones induce the pain response. The headache may actually be protecting you or warning you of something damaging, just like if you touch something hot or sharp you feel the pain and pull away so not to get burned or cut.

Any type of hormone introduced into the body may cause a headache. Hormones such as oral contraceptives, birth control patches and hormone replacement therapy can cause a hormone headache. A hormone headache can also occur at the start of, during or immediately after a period or during ovulation.

In women, hormones are not the only trigger; it is also the serotonin that interacts with the unique hormones of women. Menstrual migraines are mainly caused by estrogen. When the estrogen and progesterone levels change we are more vulnerable to headaches.

There are usually two types of hormonal headaches: Menstrual and premenstrual (or PMS) headache.

A menstrual headache generally starts one to two days prior to when the period begins or during ovulation and subsides on the second or third day. In some cases the headaches will start one to two days after your period has ended.

A premenstrual or PMS headache starts before your period and is associated with a variety of symptoms such as headache pain, fatigue, acne, decreased urination and lack of coordination. You may also experience increased appetite and a craving for chocolate, sweets, something salty or alcohol.

A minimal percentage of woman in their childbearing years suffer from migraines. In most cases, pregnancy protects a woman from migraines because the hormones remain fairly consistent throughout pregnancy. Women do not get menses so there isn't a fluctuation of hormones. If a woman suffers from a migraine during pregnancy it will generally subside after the first trimester. I myself recall having severe migraines during my first trimester and because I was pregnant I was unable to take anything to help me with the pain. I remember being awake for hours throughout the night pacing because of the pain. For the most part they did subside after the first trimester.

If you are pregnant and still experiencing migraines you should not take any medications however if you do be careful what you take. During the first trimester the baby is the most susceptible to drug-induced problems. Your doctor may prescribe medications at any point in pregnancy. Just be caution and weight the decision seriously. There are therapies that should be considered which are not chemically induces. After delivery it is common for a new mother to experience headache. If you are nursing you will still need to be careful what medications you are taking as most drugs are found to secrete in breast milk. Always check with a doctor.

Rebound, Sinus and Other Headaches

Anyone can get a rebound headache. What is a rebound headache? Well as my doctor described to me, a rebound headache occurs when you overuse either prescribed or OTC analgesic medications. When these types of medications are used on a daily or near daily basis they can be responsible for starting the headache process.

The medication may decrease the severity of the headache for a few hours but it feeds into the pain system in a way that chronic headaches could occur. For example: say you have a horrible migraine and you take Excedrin or Fioricet and two to three hours later your headache comes back stronger. That is a rebound headache. You would probably take another dose of the medicine. This cycle will continue until the analgesic medication is completely out of your system. Once you have discontinued this medication you may experience a more severe headache, nausea and/or vomiting for several days while the medication is leaving your system. After about three to five days your symptoms will begin to improve.

It is hard to not reach for something that is helpful even if it is only for a couple hours. I personally preferred the Fioricet because I would wake up with a really bad migraine and have to go to work. Most of the time, the Fioricet would take enough of the edge off so I would be able to work. That particular medication does give you rebound headaches.

A rebound headache may feel like a dull, tension type headache or could be a more severe migraine like headache. Other types of medication may not be helpful while the analgesic medications are being over used. A rebound headache can occur with most analgesic but are most likely in medications containing caffeine or butalbital.

Sinus headaches are usually in your forehead bone, the check bone on one side and behind the bridge of your nose. A lot of people believe their headache is a sinus headache because of the location. The pain is usually restricted to the sinus and is made worse by sudden movements or bending over. These types of headaches generally occur when your sinuses become inflamed usually by allergies, or an infection.

If your sinuses are blocked by an infection you will probably also have a fever and your doctor will most likely prescribe you an antibiotic to treat the infection as well as antihistamines or decongestants. If you do not have a true sinus headache and take decongestants for example they could make your headache worse.

People with migraine or headaches are at a higher risk of also suffering from allergies or asthma. One common factor of both disorders is inflammation. There are some people who have respiratory or season allergies that contribute to or cause headaches starting from there nasal passages or sinuses. At times, people who suffer from migraines and other headache types may get headaches related to allergies. The allergic reaction may provoke an increase in normal headaches. Some migraine or headache sufferers will experience nasal congestion or sinus type symptoms as part of the headache attack. These should not be confused with sinus headaches or a sinus infection. A doctor can diagnose and treat these headaches.

A silent migraine is one name for a migraine without headache pain. This may sound strange but it is not all that unusual. There have been several different names for this type of migraine such as migraine aura without headache, sans-migraine, eye migraine, and visual migraine to name a few.

A silent migraine or migraine aura without headache usually occurs later in life and generally more in men than in women. Migraine aura is a term used to describe many of the symptoms that occur with this type of headache but generally referring to the visual symptoms. You may experience visual disturbances such as flashing lights, zigzag's or spots. You may experience vertigo or dizziness. Some of the warning signs that you may experience are slurred speech, numbness, pain in other parts of your body such as your face or on the skin and/or ringing in the ears. You could experience these types of warnings with most headache types.

You could image with so many symptoms and most headaches have some if not all of the same symptoms; it is easy to be misdiagnosed. The only thing that is specifically different about this type of headache compared to other headache types is the fact that this one is missing the actual headache pain. Anyone can experience a silent migraine from time to time, even if you get another type of migraine or headache.

I personally have experience several different types of headaches. It is easier to tell what type of headache you have is you have the facts about all the headache types. Then you become aware of where the pain is and what warnings or symptoms you have before and/or during your headaches. You could feel a change in your headaches which is scary. You will usually be sent for more scans and test when there is a change in headache. It is more likely that you have developed a different type of headache.

For example say you are used to having the pain in the back of your head and neck as well as your forehead or temple (migraine), the pain is usually a throbbing pain. Then one day you wake up with a headache that feels like a vise around your temples and forehead and it is a dull pain and there is pressure (tension headache). You are just experiencing a different headache. Perhaps something is going on in your life that is causing you stress or anxiety. The key for dealing with any headache type is to recognize the type and all changes with your headache. A neurologist will have you use a headache diary. This is helpful for them as well as you.

Another type of headache is an Organic headache. An organic headache is the result of an abnormality in the brain or skull. It is generally caused by a tumor, a brain aneurysm, hematoma, meningitis, brain abscess, brain infection, cerebral hemorrhage or encephalitis. There are a very small percentage of headaches caused by tumors, not everyone with a tumor will experience a headache. A tumor will cause a headache if it intrudes on an artery or increases intracranial pressure. If there is a brain tumor, the headache will probably come on suddenly and be intense.

Some symptoms that can be a red flag are a sudden sharp, intense pain (particularly if you never or rarely have a headache); sudden lack of balance or falling; confusion; difficulty speaking; inappropriate behavior and seizures. It is imperative to seek medical assistance immediately.

Some people will experience a migraines attack during the middle of the night or in the early morning. This is considered a nocturnal migraine. This type of migraine often awakens people from their sleep. Recently it has been found that these types of attacks are related to changes in the neurotransmitters in the brain during sleep. If possible, treat the headache when the attack begins, elevate your upper torso (back, shoulders and head) and try to rest or go back to sleep.

New daily persistent headache (NDPH) is described as the rapid development of an unrelenting headache. Many people who suffer from this type of headache know exactly when the headache began and have experienced daily headaches since that time.

NDPH generally occurs in people with no past history of headache. It does not evolve from a migraine or episodic tension headache but begins as a new headache. There is some evidence that supports it may be caused by a viral infection. The symptoms for this type of headache are similar to migraine and tension type headaches whereas the person may experience sensitivity to light and/or sound, mild nausea and mild to moderate non-throbbing pain on both sides of the head.

Migraine equivalents are considered a migraine in a form other than head pain. This is generally diagnosed by determining if there is a previous history of migraine attacks, no evidence of an organic migraine, no physical lesions and the replacement of a normal headache but with the headache symptoms. It is important to be thoroughly checked out by a physician and make sure the physician is aware of any past or family history of migraine. Generally the same medication used to treat migraine is helpful with this type of migraine.

Although this is a rare type of migraine, the most common migraine equivalent is an abdominal migraine. An abdominal migraine has episodes of vomiting and abdominal pain without the headache pain. They can last for hours and occur most frequently in female children. Symptoms can show as yawning, listlessness and drowsiness during the attack. Other types of symptoms that may be experienced are visual symptoms such as blind spots, partial vision disturbances or psychic disturbances without headache pain.

Exertion headaches are associated with physical activity. They typically become severe very quickly after strenuous activity such as running, coughing, sneezing, sexual intercourse, and exerting yourself while exercising. In some cases, this type of headache may be a sign of an abnormality in the brain.

WEATHER AND HEADACHES

Another contributing factor for most headache sufferers is the weather. I can always tell when it is raining or about to rain because I begin to feel pressure in my head and my headache will get worse. Even if I recently took something to help the pain, it will intensify my existing headache.

I worked in an office where the room I worked in didn't have any windows. It could be a beautiful day outside when I went out at lunch and an hour later I could tell you that it was raining or was about to rain. My co-workers thought I was better than the meteorologist. This is caused by a change in the barometric pressure brought in by any weather front. Even cold fronts can cause a headache. It's really no different than people who have arthritis that are in more pain when it is cold or raining.

Heat and humidity can also cause or worsen a headache. You may or may not realize it but weather plays a huge role. I live in Florida. We have a constant change in pressure during hurricane season; back and forth pressure changes with cold fronts and warm fronts during the fall and winter seasons and the intense heat and humidity during the summer making the weather a mitigating factor in regards to headaches.

I read about a study by researchers at Jefferson Medical College in Philadelphia in regards to the weather and migraine sufferers. The study was performed with migraine sufferers and "normal" individuals and they compared their reaction to weather changes. It was found that migraines are more likely when the pressure rises and in some cases when the temperature rises as well. It is believed that it is not the pressure alone that causes the migraine but a variety of weather factors that trigger migraine.

According to another study done in the early eighty's they found that during "Phase four" weather migraines increase. Phase four is described as weather with low pressure, a passage of a warm front, high temperatures, humidity and often the sky is overcast. According to the American Headache Foundation changes in weather can cause the chemicals in your body to change which is another factor that can also trigger migraines. You can go to www.weather.com; they have a forecast for "aches and pains" which is based on the dropping in pressure, increased humidity and extreme temperature changes.

There isn't anything we can do about the weather. At least with headaches attributed to the weather we can get some sort of warning with weather forecasts. You can also try ionizers and humidifiers but that will not completely solve the problem.

Children and Headaches

If you are a parent or relative of a child who has headaches it can truly break your heart. Whenever you see a child, especially your own, in pain of any kind all you want to do is make it better. So when you have a child who gets headaches or migraines you, in a sense, suffer along with your child. You may not experience the physical pain your child is feeling but not being able to make it better is disheartening in its own right.

If you are a parent of a child that gets headaches and you yourself get them then it can be even worse as you know *exactly* what your child is feeling. You have a deeper understanding since you also go through this. Then you begin to wonder if it is hereditary and if your child is going to have to deal with this their entire life.

It isn't abnormal for a child to start getting headaches in adolescence since there are hormonal changes we all go through. There are a lot of things that can cause headaches in children. Headaches are a frequent symptom in children, it is finding out whether or not it is related to something else that can be difficult. It is first necessary to bring your child to a doctor so they can figure out the type of headache your child is having. Then they can go about finding the correct way to treat the headache.

Doctors determine the types of headache by the placement of the pain and the symptoms that are being experienced. This is not the root cause of a headache just the way to determine the type of headache. It is important for the doctor to have a full and accurate history in order to make a diagnosis. It is also important that the doctor speak with the child with the parents as well as without the parents. This way the doctor can see how the parent and child interact and also give the child an opportunity to discuss things they may not want to say in front of their parent.

Children's headaches can be classified as they are in adults: Migraine, tension and organic.

Tension type – This is the most common type of headache in children. As previously mention in the chapter on tension headaches, the pain associated with this type of headache is tightening in the muscles especially around the neck and usually is not accompanied by vomiting or nausea. Your child's tension headache is most commonly caused by poor posture, worry, anxiety or depression.

Migraine –The blood vessels and arteries in and around the skull expand causing swelling which applies pressure to the nerves which cause pain. The pain is generally a throbbing pain and almost always come with nausea and vomiting. In children, the headache is often on both sides of the head instead on just one side. Children may appear to be pale or have glassy eyes, and may be irritable before or during the attack. If the child gets periodic vomiting without the migraine or exhibit car or motion sickness this may be an indication that at some point they may develop migraines, especially if there is a family history of them. Migraine may occur after a head injury, especially after an injury related to sport activities such as football, soccer, baseball or hockey.

Organic headache – This type usually indicates the presence of some type of abnormality such as a tumor, abscess, infection, swelling or hematoma. If a new or sudden headache with fever, weakness or exhaustion and a stiff neck occur consult a doctor immediately. A doctor can spot these abnormalities on the scans (MRI, MRA, CAT scan or X-ray). This is considered an organic headache. These types of headaches require immediate medical care. Other symptoms include nausea, vomiting, lack of coordination, seizures and personality changes.

Some of the causes of headache in children are:

Inflammation – When the tissues are irritated or injured they become inflamed meaning swollen. An inflammation headache might be accompanied by diseases of the eyes, ears, nose, teeth or sinuses, neck or jaw disorders. This is also considered an organic type of headache and requires immediate medical care. Note inflammation of the blood vessels often occurs with headaches. When inflammation of the tissue occurs it can cause a different type of headache and a doctor should be consulted.

Stress – Children can experience stress, anxiety and depression as adults do. This can cause a headache in children. Something stressful may be occurring in your child's life that is causing him or her to worry or become depressed. Something at school could be the cause such as bullying or worrying about grades or your child may be depressed due to changes or something going on at home.

Hunger- Your child's headache may be as simple as he or she is hungry. If, after a full night's sleep and your child hasn't eaten breakfast or lunch he or she may be suffering from a hunger headache. The treatment would be breakfast, something with bread or a fiber-rich cereal and milk. Encourage your child to eat a mid-morning snack such as fruit and a good lunch.

Physical strain – In this day and age it would be common for your child to suffer from eye strain. With all the technology; video games, iPad, iPod, TV or even if your child is a reader and has to strain their eyes to read the words. The headache could also be the cause of neck or back strain or by poor posture.

Food and diet – Food and diet can definitely trigger headaches and migraines. In a later chapter we will go over different foods both good and bad for headaches.

In some cases, children tend to have fewer headaches after they are reassured that there are no abnormalities. Having regular routines such as bedtimes and good eating habits at the same time of day are beneficial. Make sure your child drinks a lot of fluids especially when outside playing in hot or humid weather for an extended amount of time or during exercise so they do not get dehydrated as well. Limit the amount of caffeine and sugar they have. Try monitoring the amount of time your child spends reading, doing school work or playing video games and watching TV. In children younger than 12 years old with infrequent attacks, try children's Tylenol or Motrin. If your child gets migraine type headaches a doctor may be able to prescribe something to help prevent and maintain migraines. It is important that your child's school is aware of the headaches. Your child's doctor should work together with your child's school to make sure that treatment is available at the onset of a headache. Children respond well to biofeedback.

Exercise and Migraines

I know when you have a migraine activity makes it worse. There has been many time I wanted to go to the gym or throw the football around with my son but couldn't. There are so many activities that you become limited from because of the pain. It's not that regular exercise is a trigger but the movement alone can increase the migraine you have. Strenuous exercise can cause a headache but it is said that moderate aerobic exercise can be therapeutic, help decrease the migraines and possibly prevent an attack.

Studies have shown that exercise changes the levels of a wide range of your body's chemicals. Exercise stimulates endorphins which are a natural pain controlling chemical. Exercise also releases encephalin which is a natural anti-depressant. It is very possible that if you have a regular exercise routine you could reduce the amount of headaches you get as well as the severity of the headaches, you could also reduce your drug intake especially the drugs taken daily. You may not need them as much.

You may have found that exercise is one of your triggers. That may be due to the following reasons:

- ❖ You start exercising suddenly without warming up and getting your body ready for the change. You could have a lack of oxygen because your body is just not ready yet.
- ❖ You may not be eating properly prior to exercising causing your blood sugar to drop and you become very hunger.

Perhaps you are not drinking plenty of fluids and you are dehydrated.

❖ You may be starting too much at once. For example, you begin a new healthy diet and at the same time start a "fit" exercise program. It's not that those are bad things, both are very good and important, you just have to be careful and manage them properly. Don't do too much too quick. This can be a shock to your body and act as a trigger.

❖ You start a strenuous infrequent workout routine which leaves your muscles stiff and sore for days which can act as a trigger.

❖ Exercise may act as a trigger during the exercise itself (called an exertion headache) which generally occurs at high altitudes or during hot weather. This may last from five minutes to forty-eight hours.

Make sure you choose the right exercise for you. Mild aerobic exercise offers the most benefits to people who suffer from migraine. Choose something that you enjoy like swimming, jogging, dancing, walking or cycling.

When you first start a new exercise routine try to avoid strenuous or competitive activities until you are more accustomed to exercising and are more in shape. Try to exercise at least thirty minutes at moderate intensity a few times a week and give yourself at least six weeks to see if there is any beneficial changes. See if your local gym offers short aerobic or dance classes such as Zumba or even a cycling class. Most gyms have trainers that you can ask questions. Have someone help to see what exercises would be best for you. If you prefer not to go to a gym, maybe you and a friend could walk briskly or go to the park and throw a football back and forth. Playing tennis and swimming are also good options. You could join a local community center (such as a YMCA). Get your heart rate up some.

Preparing to exercise is just as important as the exercise itself. You should begin an exercise program gradually, building up momentum over several weeks. Start with short sessions and gradually go longer but be careful not to over exert yourself in the process.

Make sure you eat an hour to an hour and a half prior to exercising. This way your body can digest the food and eating prior to exercise helps to avoid low blood sugar which can trigger a headache.

Make sure to drink a lot of fluids prior to, during and after exercise. You lose fluid while exercising from sweating. If you do not drink plenty of fluids you can become dehydrated. This is a major trigger for migraines. You should always have a bottle of water or a sport drink such as Gatorade readily available. You could also drink isotonic drinks which are found in health food stores. These will keep your body in balance.

You should never start or stop exercising suddenly. Stretch for about five to ten minutes at the beginning and the end of exercising. The warm up and cool down are important to preparing your body and preventing muscle tension.

Make sure to dress accordingly. Wear the correct shoes and light, loose, comfortable clothing. If you ever begin to feel uncomfortable start the cool down and then stop.

Make sure to keep track of your exercise routine in your headache diary. This will help to keep track of the affects the exercise is having. Make note of the date and time, your warm up, the type of exercises and the length of time. List all medications you are taking, what you have eaten and drank and whether or not you've experienced a headache or if you had one if it improved or had become worse.

Diet and Headaches

In most cases, foods and drinks can be a trigger for headaches and migraines. There are certain types of foods and beverages you should avoid. Keep in mind though, not every person who experience migraine or headache has a dietary trigger. There are some common foods and beverages that are known to trigger headaches and migraine for the sufferer. This is another way keeping a headache journal would be very useful.

Try to avoid nitrates or nitrites. They are generally found in certain types of heart medications, and used as a preservative in some foods and beverages. Nitrites are used to preserve the red coloring in processed meats such as hot dogs, bologna, salami, bacon, etc.

Tyramine is naturally produced in foods. It is important to those who have food triggers to have a low tyramine diet. Tyramine levels increase in foods that are aged, fermented or foods that are not fresh.

Meats, poultry, fish and eggs: Try to eat freshly purchased and prepared. Be caution when using bacon, sausage, hot dogs, corned beef and any lunch meat that has nitrates or nitrites added. Avoid aged, dried, fermented, salted, smoked or pickled products such as salami, pepperoni and liverwurst.

Dairy: Drinking or using whole, 2% or skim milk is fine. Cheeses such as American, cottage, ricotta, cream cheese, Velveeta and low-fat processed cheeses are all okay. Be careful when eating or using yogurt, sour cream, Parmesan and Romano cheeses. Try to avoid aged cheeses such as blue, brick, brie, Swiss, cheddar, mozzarella, provolone, etc.

Breads and pasta: Commercially prepared yeasts are good but try to avoid homemade yeast breads and coffee cake. Breads made with baking power are all okay. All cooked and dry cereals and all pastas are okay as well.

Vegetables: Be careful with raw onion and try to avoid fermented products such as soy sauce, teriyaki sauce, snow peas, sauerkraut, pickles and olives. Vegetables such as asparagus, string beans, carrots, spinach, zucchini, broccoli, potatoes, and cooked onions are all fine to eat.

Soups made from fresh ingredients are all fine but try to avoid canned soups, bouillon bases and soups containing autolytic yeasts or that which contain MSG.

Fruits: Be cautious with citrus, orange, pineapple, tangerine, and grapefruit; try to limit to half a cup per day. Also be careful when eating avocado, banana, figs, raisins, papaya, red plums, and passion fruit. Apples, cherries, apricots, and peaches are fine to eat.

Nuts and seeds: Try to avoid all nuts. Peanuts, peanut butter, walnuts, and pecans, pumpkin seeds, sunflower seed and sesame seeds.

Beverages: It's okay to drink decaffeinated beverages, caffeine- free carbonated sodas, and fruit juices. Try to limit yourself with caffeinated beverages. Too much caffeine can cause a headache. Limit alcohol; Riesling wine, vodka or scotch are okay to drink in moderation. Try to avoid red wines, Chianti, sherry, burgundy, vermouth, ale, beer, and non-alcoholic fermented beverages.

Desserts: Be careful eating chocolate based products. This may not be what women want to hear.

Miscellaneous: Avoid products containing NutraSweet, aspartame, and MSG. These have a tendency to trigger headaches and migraines.

This is just a guide of certain foods and drinks that have ingredients that have been found to trigger headaches in some people. Remember everyone is different, some may find that very few or none of the foods trigger a headache and some of you may find that many of them do. I suggest testing the ones you wish and track the results in your headache diary.

TRIGGERS

There are various factors that can trigger a headache. In order to avoid what may trigger your headache you must first identify what your triggers are. Keeping a headache journal or diary can play a crucial role in identifying your triggers. Keeping a headache diary is not hard to do. My headache diary is a mini composition notebook. You should track how many hours you sleep, describe any stressful events that occur, note the time your headache begins and the duration of the headache, what medication, dosage and how often you took the medication. Also note if your headache has improved or if it has become worse.

No two people are exactly the same. Even identical twins have differences. One twin may be more cautious while the other has a wild, adventurous side. They may look the same but they are in fact different. We are like snowflakes, each beautifully unique. So why would our headaches or any aspect of our headaches be the same.

The best way to figure out what triggers your headache is when you notice you have a headache think back to what you did right before it started. Did you just eat something? Were you reading, jogging, did it start raining or does it look like it is about to rain?

First identify your triggers then if possible avoid what you have found to trigger them. I noticed that when I eat dark chocolate I get a headache but milk chocolate or white chocolate do not affect me.

Some triggers you will have no control over such as the weather. Control the ones you can, that is a good start at a life with less pain.

I have listed some of the most common triggers.

Dietary triggers: Foods containing MSG such as some Chinese foods or nitrites which are contained in hot dogs and other processed meats. Pickled foods containing tyramine, aged cheeses, excessive caffeine, chocolate, fermented foods and dried or smoked foods. Try to avoid alcoholic beverages, especially red wine. Alcohol, which is found in beverages such as liquor, beer and wine, has a chemical called Ethanol. Ethanol causes headaches in a variety of ways. It is a direct vasodilator. In some people vasodilatation causes headaches. Ethanol is also a natural diuretic. Excessive consumption of Ethanol may cause dehydration and other chemical imbalances in the body which may cause headaches.

Environmental triggers: Secondhand smoke, bright light, perfume or strong odors and weather changes. Any changes in a migraine or headache sufferer's environment can trigger a headache; whether it is changing jobs or schools, travelling, being in a stuffy room or flying in an airplane. There are many environmental factors that can trigger a headache.

Lifestyle triggers: Excessive stress, physical exertion, missing meals and lack of sleep. Try going to bed and waking up the same time every day. Too much or too little sleep can be a trigger. Smoking is also a trigger for headaches both for the smoker as well as the nonsmoker. Nicotine has vascular effects which can trigger a headache in those susceptible to headache. This is most evident in those who get tension headaches.

Hormonal triggers: Onset of puberty, menstruation, menopause, pregnancy, birth control pills, and hormone replacement therapy.

Herbal Treatments

There are a lot of different treatments for headaches and migraines. The effectiveness of the treatment is dependent upon the headache type and the person being treated. What I mean by that is, for example, a combination such as Feverfew (herb), Magnesium (mineral) and Vitamin B taken daily may work on one individual and have no effect at all on another. I would hear someone talk about a specific type of medication or treatment that worked well for them or read about another treatment and was at the point I would try just about anything since I hadn't had much luck so far. The trick is to find what works for you. A chiropractor may be very effective for one person and make the pain worse for another. Don't give up, you can find something or a combination of things that are effective for you.

With all herbs and medications, always use as directed. Using too much could result in rebound headaches and dependency issues or worse. Even though it may be an herb, there are healing properties and some are just as potent or unsafe as some chemical medications. Some people are under the misconception that it's an herb and natural therefore they could take however much they want in order to obtain their desired effect. When or if you wish to discontinue using either herbs or medications the best way to discontinue is to gradually wean or reduce your dosage until you have completely stopped taking it. A doctor can safely assist you. You can find the below referenced herbs where vitamins and herbal supplements are sold or where loose and bulk herbs are sold (including mail-order). My favorite website for herbs is www.mountainroseherbs.com

BUTTERBUR:

Butterbur has anti-inflammatory, anti-allergenic and antispasmodic properties. The root is the part of the plant that is used. Butterbur has been shown to reduce the frequency, duration and intensity of migraine attacks. This is also safe to give to children six years old and older suffering from migraine at an advised dose. Butterbur is to be taken in a standardized extract. The wild plant, not the extract, is toxic to the liver. Do not take while pregnant or nursing. Rarely, may cause gastrointestinal upset or drowsiness. This herb is restricted in some countries.

CAYENNE:

Cayenne has anti-inflammatory, anti-irritant, anti-fungal, anti-cold-flu, and anti-allergen properties as well as others. The part of the plant used is the pepper (or fruit) and the seeds. Cayenne contains vitamins A and C along with the alkaloid capsaicin. Capsaicin is a powerful stimulant and irritant. Capsaicin is an ingredient found in many kinds of peppers which among other things raises your pain threshold. Capsaicin triggers nerves repeatedly, causing pain at first. Afterwards, pain signals can no longer be sent. Cayenne also can be used to dilate blood vessels, improving blood flow. These effects are all temporary, but happen immediately. Cayenne is considered safe but not recommended for children under two years old.

COFFEE:

Coffee is a diuretic and stimulant. The part used is the bean. It's not too much of a stretch to think coffee would be helpful with migraine or headache. A lot of migraine medications have caffeine in them and coffee is caffeine. A steaming hot cup of coffee could definitely be helpful in alleviating a headache or migraine. However, excessive use of coffee may also cause a headache or migraine as with excessive use of anything with caffeine. Coffee is considered safe; avoid excessive amounts which can cause palpitations.

FEVERFEW:

Feverfew is the most commonly known herb used to help migraine and tension headaches. This is an anti-inflammatory herb and the leaves of the plant are what are used. It is helpful at the first signs that a migraine is coming. When taken daily may be helpful in reducing the amount of or the severity of migraines. It doesn't work well as a rescue medication for full-blown migraines. You will receive the best results when used on a regular basis. When taking long term use caution when discontinuing as you can induce withdrawal symptoms.

Do not take more than recommended unless directed by a doctor. This herb is considered generally safe when taken as recommended. The possible side effects of Feverfew include nausea, vomiting and diarrhea. If the herb is chewed it may cause mouth ulcers and swelling/numbness of the mouth. Do not take if you are pregnant or nursing. Feverfew may interact with medications such as blood thinners and liver metabolizing medications.

LAVENDER:

Lavender has analgesic, antiseptic, sedative and antidepressant properties. The leaf, flowers and essential oils are the parts of the plant uses. Lavender is useful for headache, anxiety, irritability, sleep, and pain relief (and others not listed). Lavender is probably best known for its calming qualities. A cup of lavender tea prior to bed will assist with falling asleep. You can also put some essential oil in an oil burner and this will also help with falling asleep or relaxing. Lavender has mood-enhancing qualities since it has a nature combination of antidepressant and mild sedative properties. The relaxing qualities are also known to help alleviate tension or stress headaches. An essential oil of Lavender can be applied to the skin in almost any situation regarding pain. If you have a headache you can apply the essential oil to the temples and forehead to ease the pain. Lavender is helpful for many different things aside from headaches. It is a safe herb. Do not ingest the essential oil.

PASSION FLOWER:

Passion flower aids in sleep; is a relaxant, relieves pain and has sedative properties. It is considered safe, non-addictive and rarely produces drowsiness. The aerial parts are what are used on the plant. This is a good herb for relieving stress and anxiety as well as tension headache. It has a mild analgesic which is helpful in relieving migraines and neuralgic pain associated with toothaches.

PEPPERMINT:

Peppermint has mild sedative, mild analgesic, antiseptic and antispasmodic properties. The leaves and the essential oil are what are used from the plant. Peppermint is helpful with migraine and headaches as well as the nausea which sometimes accompanies headache and migraine. You may drink an infusion of peppermint tea or use the essential oil by applying 1-2 drops to your forehead. Also effective is to rub a drop of the essential oil under your nose as the smell helps with not only the headache but also nausea. Be careful not to use too much of the essential oil as it will be too strong and may intensify the headache. Peppermint is considered safe. Do not give to children under the age of five.

ROSEMARY:

This is an anti-inflammatory, antispasmodic, antioxidant and stimulates circulation. It's also considered a tonic for nerves and digestion. The leaf is the part of the plant that is uses as well as the essential oil. An infusion of Rosemary can bring quick relief to nervous or tension headaches. If you have a headache that is linked to high blood pressure, combine Rosemary with *Linden flowers*. It is also helpful with migraine.

Rosemary is considered generally safe but can cause and allergic skin reaction when used in topical preparations. Best used as an infusion, tincture or essential oil. Rosemary is often used with Lavender. Avoid consuming large quantities when pregnant or nursing.

WILLOW BARK:

Willow is nature's aspirin. Do not use if you have an allergy or sensitivity to aspirin or if you need to avoid aspirin due to medications you are currently taking. Also do not take willow with aspirin. One of aspirins active ingredients is acetylsalicylic acid, which is a chemical derivative of salicin, a natural pain reliever found in several plants.

Willow has antioxidant, fever reducing, antiseptic, and immune boosting properties. Since Willow has some of the same properties as aspirin you should use the same cautions. Do not use while pregnant or nursing. Do not use for children without first speaking with a doctor. If you are not sure whether it is safe for you to take Willow, check with your doctor prior to using.

Prescription Rescue Medications

In this section we will go over some of the most common prescription medications for headaches and migraines. There are two categories that medications are prescribed. The first category is abortive or rescue medications. These are medications used to treat individual migraine or headache attacks. The second category is for preventative medications. This type of medication is used on an ongoing basis to reduce headache severity and frequency.

There is a large variety of medications used for headaches and migraines. Many are prescribed for other medical issues and have been found helpful for headaches and migraines. Not every medication will work for every individual. More likely than not, it will take several attempts to find the correct medication and dosage or combination of medications that will be effective for you. There isn't a *cure* for migraines only treatments to improve them.

Don't get discouraged if you don't find your remedy tomorrow or next week. There are a lot of options even though it doesn't feel like it right now. I understand that when you are in pain you just want the pain to end; the sooner the better. Remember the severity of the pain when you start each treatment; write the details in your headache journal. At some point go back, read what you wrote down and remember how you felt at the beginning and compare it to how you feel with each change in your treatment. This will help you notice what is helpful and what is not. It will take baby steps, at some point you will find something that helps, and then you and your doctor can build on that.

Make sure all your doctors have a current list of everything you are taking including any herbal and vitamin supplements.

While researching the medication section of this book, I used several accurate websites. Accurate information regarding prescription drugs is *extremely important* so there isn't an interaction or reaction that could lead to a more serious issue. As not to make an error with any of the valuable and important information regarding medications, I have found the vast majority of this information from the reputable sites listed below. You can find further information on these sites if there is something not mentioned or if you want to further research any medications yourself.

National Center for Biotechnology Information, U.S. National Library of Medicine at www.ncbi.nlm.nih.gov
Walgreens at www.walgreens.com
National Headache Foundation at www.headaches.org

Medications are listed by the generic name and the brand name associated.
The first and one of the most commonly used medication for migraine headaches is the triptan family of medications. Triptan medications are a class of medications called selective serotonin receptor agonists. Triptans are used to treat the symptoms of migraine headaches (severe, throbbing headaches that sometimes are accompanied by nausea and sensitivity to sound and light). It works by narrowing blood vessels in the brain, stopping pain signals from being sent to the brain, and stopping the release of certain natural substances that cause

pain, nausea, and other symptoms of migraine. Triptan medications do not prevent migraine attacks.

Common side effects that may occur include dizziness; drowsiness; dry mouth; fatigue; flushing; headache; hot or cold sensations; indigestion; numbness or tingling in the arms, legs, hands, or feet.

ALMOTRIPTAN-AXERT.

ELETRIPTAN-RALPAX

FROVATRIPTAN-FROVA

NARATRIPTAN-AMERGE

RIZATRIPTAN-MAXALT

SUMATRIPTAN-IMITREX

ZOLMITRIPTAN-ZOMIG

The next class of medications is ergotamine. Ergot alkaloids, ergotamine tartrate (ET) and dihydroergotamine (DHE) are effective therapies for migraine and cluster headache. This type of medication stimulates serotonin, decreases inflammation and reverses blood vessel dilation around the brain relieving the migraine or cluster headache symptoms.

ERGOT ALKALOID: BELLERGAL-S, BELLAMINE, CAFFERGOT, ERGOSTAT, DIHYDROERGOTAMINE (also known as D.H.E. 45 Injection), MIGRANAL (nasal spray), and METHYSERGIDE (also known as SANSERT).

For the best results with these medications several factors must be taken into account, including headache type and severity, associated symptoms, side effect sensitivity, choice of dosage forms (such as injection, pill form or nasal spray) and correct dosage.

Oral ergotamine is an effective treatment of cluster headaches and slowly developing migraine without early onset nausea or vomiting. Ergotamine tartrate given via rectal suppository (which is only available in combination with caffeine) is the most effective form, especially for patients with severe, rapid onset migraine accompanied by nausea and/or vomiting.

Dihydroergotamine offers numerous benefits compared to ergotamine tartrate, including a lower frequency of nausea, vomiting and headache recurrence and does not cause rebound headache.

Dihydroergotamine can be used at any time during a migraine attack, including the aura phase. Intravenous administration can be done at a hospital for people with intractable severe headache (status migraines, transformed migraine, and rebound headache) and cluster headache. Intramuscularly injection is effective for moderate to severe migraine with or without nausea and vomiting.

Intranasal (nasal spray form) DHE is an effective and convenient therapy in acute migraine and may also be useful with nausea and vomiting. When used correctly, DHE and ergotamine tartrate are effective for people with migraine or cluster headaches. The most common side effects with ergotamine are nausea or vomiting.

METHYLERGONOVINE MALEATE: also called METHYLERGOBASIN and METHERGINE

Methergine is the brand name for methylergonovine maleate. Originally used for the treatment of postpartum bleeding. Methergine also causes constriction of the muscles in the blood vessels. This vasoconstriction action makes methergine helpful to some headache patients. It can be helpful in treating vascular headaches, such as migraine including menstrual migraine as well as cluster headaches. It is more commonly used for prevention of headaches, but can be taken for acute attacks. Because of the vasoconstriction effects, Methergine is used for approximately six month and then a resting period of approximately one month and only under careful of a physician.

ERGOTAMINE & CAFFEINE: MIGERGOT
 This ergot/caffeine combination works by preventing blood vessels in the head from expanding and causing headaches.

Let next discuss non-steroidal anti-inflammatory drugs also known as NSAIDS. NSAIDS are a very common and very useful pain reliever. There is a lot of OTC NSAID medications you may or may not realize is a NSAID such as Excedrin which is a combination NSAID, caffeine and acetaminophen. You need to be careful with NSAIDS. Read the label carefully as they interact with other medications. You may also develop stomach irritation or pain if used too often or excessively. Generally your doctor will prescribe or suggest a medication to take while using NSAIDs to avoid stomach irritation such as Prilosec.

Here is a list of some NSAIDS.

IB PROFEN: ADDAPRIN, ADVIL, CAP-PROFEN, COUNTERACT IB, DOLGESIC, GENPRIL, HALTAN, IBIFON 600, IBREN, IBU-TAB, IBUPROHM, MIDOL,MENADOL, MOTRIN, NUPRIN, Q-PROFEN, RUFEN, RX-ACT IBUPROFEN, SALETO, SAMSON 8, SUP PAIN MED, TAB-PROFEN, ULTRAPRIN, UNI-PRO, WAL-PROFEN

Side effects associated include constipation, diarrhea, gas or bloating, dizziness, nervousness, ringing in the ears.

Prescription ibuprofen is used to relieve pain, tenderness, swelling, and stiffness. It is also used to relieve mild to moderate pain, including menstrual pain. Nonprescription ibuprofen is used to reduce fever and to relieve mild pain from headaches, muscle aches, arthritis, menstrual periods, the common cold, toothaches, and backaches. It works by stopping the body's production of a substance that causes pain, fever, and inflammation.

DICLOFENAC POTASSIUM: CAMBIA, CATAFLAM; VOLTAREN; VOLTAROL; ZIPSOR.

Common side effects associated include nausea and dizziness.

Cambia is an oral solution you mix into water and drink. It does not prevent or lessen the number of migraines you have, and it is not for other types of headaches. It should be used at the lowest dose possible and for the shortest time needed.

KETAPROFEN: ORUDIS, ACTRON, ORUVAIL

Side effects that may go away during treatment include nausea, vomiting, diarrhea, gas, constipation, indigestion, dizziness, lightheadedness, drowsiness, nervousness, or headache.

Prescription Ketoprofen is used to relieve pain, tenderness, swelling, and stiffness. Prescription ketoprofen capsules are also used to relieve pain, including menstrual pain. Nonprescription ketoprofen is used to relieve minor aches and pain from headaches, menstrual periods, toothaches, the common cold, muscle aches, and backaches, and to reduce fever. It works by stopping the body's production of a substance that causes pain, fever, and inflammation.

KETOROLAC: TORADOL

Side effects that may occur during treatment include constipation; diarrhea; dizziness; drowsiness; gas; headache; indigestion; mild stomach pain or upset; nausea; pain at the injection site; stomach fullness; sweating; or vomiting.

This medicine comes as an intramuscular injection or a tablet taken by mouth used for short-term (up to 5 days) treatment of moderately severe pain alone or in combination with other medicines. Do not use more than five consecutive days. Using more than five days in a row may cause serious heart problems. This medication should only be used under the care of a physician.

KETOROLAC: TROMETHAMINE, SPRIX

Side effects that may occur during treatment include constipation; diarrhea; dizziness; drowsiness; gas; headache; indigestion; mild stomach pain or upset; nausea; pain at the injection site; stomach fullness; sweating; or vomiting.

This medicine is the same as above except in a nasal spray. You should also use caution with this medication and use no more than five consecutive days.

NABUMETONE: RELAFEN

Side effects that that may go away during treatment, include diarrhea or constipation, heartburn, nausea, vomiting, gas, dizziness, headache, dry mouth, or trouble sleeping

Nabumetone is used to relieve pain, tenderness, swelling, and stiffness.

NAPROXEN SODIUM: AFLAXEN, ALEVE, ANAPROX, MIDOL XR, NAPRELAN, MAPROSYN, WAL-PROXEN

Side effects that may go away during treatment include upset stomach, nausea, heartburn, gas, headache, diarrhea, constipation, drowsiness, stuffy nose, or dizziness.

Naproxen is used for temporary relief of minor aches and pains. These may include arthritis, muscle aches, backache, menstrual cramps, headache, toothache, and those due to a cold. It is also used to reduce fever.

HYDROCODONE-IBUPROF: VICOPROFEN

Side effects that may occur while taking this medicine include anxiety, constipation, diarrhea, dizziness, dry mouth, gas, headache, heartburn, increased sweating, loss of appetite, nausea, nervousness, stomach pain or upset, trouble sleeping, vomiting, and weakness.

This medicine is an analgesic and nonsteroidal anti-inflammatory drug (NSAID) combination used for short term pain relief.

SUMPATRIPTAN & NAPROXEN: TREXIMET

Side effects that may occur while taking this medicine include constipation, diarrhea, dizziness, drowsiness, gas, heartburn, mild feeling of heaviness or pressure, mild numbness or tingling of the skin, nausea, stomach upset, tiredness, or a warm or hot sensation.

This medication contains naproxen (NSAID) and sumatriptan (triptan). It is used to treat migraines when they occur. It helps to relieve headache and other symptoms of migraines, including sensitivity to light/sound, nausea, and vomiting.

The next group of drugs is Narcotic prescription medications. It is extremely important to use caution when taking this type of medication. This class of drugs is highly addictive and should only be used for a short period of time under the care of a physician. This class of drug is very effective as a rescue medication however often cause rebound headaches when taken too frequently and/or on a daily basis. There are a lot of risks associated with this type of drug. It is important to use caution and keep your doctor informed of your progress.

ACETAMINOPHEN, BUTALBITAL, CAFFEINE: ESGIC, FIORICET, FIROINOL, REPAN

Side effects that may occur include drowsiness, dizziness, lightheadedness, or nausea.

This medicine is an analgesic, barbiturate, and stimulant combination used to treat tension headaches. This combination medication is used to treat tension headaches. Acetaminophen helps to decrease the pain from the headache. Caffeine helps increase the effects of acetaminophen. Butalbital is in a group of drugs called barbiturates. It relaxes muscle contractions involved in a tension headache. Butalbital is a sedative that helps to decrease anxiety and cause sleepiness and relaxation.

ACETAMINOPHEN, BUTALBITAL: BUPAP

Side effects that may occur include headache, dizziness, drowsiness, shaky feeling; drunk feeling; vomiting, constipation; heartburn, trouble swallowing; numbness or tingly feeling; dry mouth; sweating or urinating more than usual, leg pain, tired muscles; stuffy nose, ear pain, ringing in your ears; or mild itching.

Acetaminophen is a pain reliever. Butalbital is in a group of drugs called barbiturates. It relaxes muscle contractions involved in a tension headache. Butalbital is a sedative that helps to decrease anxiety and cause sleepiness and relaxation. The combination of Bupap is used to treat tension headaches. This medicine is not for treating headaches that come and go.

BUTRANS
Side effects that may occur include constipation; dizziness; drowsiness; dry mouth; fatigue; headache; itching, rash, or redness at the application site; nausea; sweating; or vomiting.

Butrans comes in patch form This medicine is a narcotic analgesic used to manage moderate to severe chronic pain in patients who need continuous, around-the-clock narcotic pain relief for an extended period of time.

CODEINE
Codeine is found in a large variety of medications. Some people have allergic reacts that may include but not limited to vomiting.
Side effects include dizziness, lightheadedness, headache, drowsiness, mood change, nausea, vomiting, constipation, stomach ache, difficulty urinating.

Codeine is used to relieve mild to moderate pain.

ACETAMINOPHEN AND PROPOXYPHENE: DARVOCET
Side effects may include mild nausea, vomiting, upset stomach, constipation; feeling dizzy or drowsy; headache, blurred vision; or dry mouth.

Darvocet is used to relieve mild to moderate pain with or without fever.

DIHYDROCODEINE, ACETAMINOPHEN, CAFFEINE: ZERLOR, PANLOR SS, PANLOR DC, TREZIX

Side effects that may go away during treatment include dizziness, drowsiness, lightheadedness, constipation, nausea, or vomiting.

This medicine is an analgesic combination used to relieve pain

HYDROCODEINE/APAP: LORTAB, VICODIN

Side effects may include nausea, vomiting, constipation, lightheadedness, dizziness, drowsiness, flushing, or vision changes.

This medicine is a combination of a narcotic and acetaminophen used to relieve moderate to severe pain. Narcotic pain-relievers work by binding to opioid receptors in the brain and spinal cord, and acetaminophen is a pain reliever.

MEPERIDINE: DEMEROL

Side effects may include constipation, dizziness, drowsiness, flushing, lightheadedness, and loss of appetite, nausea, sweating, or vomiting.

Meperidine is used to relieve moderate to severe pain. Meperidine is a group of pain medications similar to morphine. It works by changing the way the body senses pain. Meperidine comes as a tablet and syrup to take by mouth or injection.

NALBUPHINE HYDROCHLORIDE: NUBAIN

Side effects that may occur while you are using this medicine include drowsiness, dizziness, constipation, or nausea.

This medicine is a narcotic analgesic used to treat or prevent moderate to severe pain.

OXYCODONE: DAZIDOX, ETH-OXYDOSE, ENDOCODONE, OXECTA, OXY IR, OXYCONTIN, OXYFAST, PERCOLONE, ROXICODONE

Side effects that may occur while using this medicine include drowsiness, dizziness, headache, sweating, weakness, dry mouth, nausea, vomiting, or constipation.

Oxycodone is used to relieve moderate to severe pain. It works by changing the way the brain and nervous system respond to pain. Oxycodone is also available in combination with acetaminophen (Endocet, Percocet, Roxicet, Tylox, ect.); or aspirin (Endodan, Percodan, Roxiprin, others); and ibuprofen (Combunox).

OXYMORPHONE: OPANA

Side effects that may occur while you are taking this medicine include constipation, dizziness, drowsiness, dry mouth, gas, headache, lightheadedness, nausea, or vomiting.

Oxymorphone is used to relieve moderate to severe pain. It works by changing the way the body responds to pain.

BUTORPHANOL: STADOL

Stadol comes as a nasal spray. Side effects that may go away during treatment include nausea, sleepiness, dizziness, sweating, dry mouth, headache, constipation, and trouble sleeping.

Butorphanol nasal spray is used to relieve moderate to severe pain. It works by changing the way the body senses pain.

TRAMADOL: RYZOLT, ULTRAM, RYBIX

Side effects that may occur while taking this medicine include: constipation; diarrhea; dizziness; drowsiness; dry mouth; headache; increased sweating; indigestion; mild itching; nausea; trouble sleeping; vomiting; weakness.

Tramadolis used to relieve moderate to moderately severe pain. Tramadol extended-release tablets are only used by people who are expected to need medication to relieve pain around-the-clock for a long time. It works by changing the way the body senses pain.

ISOMETHEPTENE, DICHLORALPHENAZONE, AND ACETAMINOPHEN: ALIDRIN, AMIDRINE, DURADRIN, EPIDRIN, I.D.A., ISO-ACETAZONE ISOCOM, MIDCHLOR, MIDRIN, MIGQUIN, MIGRAN-A, MIGRAPAP, MIGRATINE, MIGRAZONE, MIGREX, MITRIDE, VA-ZONE.

Dizziness may occur while using this medication.

This medicine is an analgesic, vasoconstrictor, and sedative combination used to treat migraine and tension headaches. It prevents blood vessels in your head from expanding and causing headaches.

Prescription Preventative Medications

Preventative medications are taken on a daily base to help prevent the occurrence and severity of migraines and headaches.

Some of the medications used for migraine prevention are beta-blockers, calcium-channel blockers, antidepressants, antipsychotic and anticonvulsant. Here is some of the more commonly known preventative medications used for migraines and headaches.

Let's begin with anti-depressant types such as SNRI (Serotonin-Norepinephrine Reuptake Inhibitor) and tricyclic antidepressants. Be sure to discuss with your doctor when attempting to stop taking antidepressants. It is important to be weaned off of these types of medication.

DESVENLAFAXINE: PRESTIQ
Side effects that may occur while taking this medicine include constipation, decreased sexual desire or ability, diarrhea, dizziness, drowsiness, dry mouth, fatigue, flushing, headache, increased sweating, loss of appetite, nausea, stomach upset, trouble sleeping, vomiting, or yawning.

Desvenlafaxine is a SNRI antidepressant used in the treatment of depression. It works by restoring the balance of natural substances in the brain. Desvenlafaxine may improve your mood, feelings of well-being, and energy level.

DOXEPIN: SINEQUAN, ADAPIN, SILENOR

Side effects that may occur include dry mouth, drowsiness, dizziness, headache, nausea, weakness, diarrhea, excess sweating, heartburn, unpleasant taste, weight gain, or an increased appetite especially for sweets.

This medicine is a tricyclic antidepressant used to treat depression.

DULOXETINE: CYMBALTA

Side effects that may occur include constipation, decreased sexual desire or ability, diarrhea, dizziness, drowsiness, dry mouth, headache, increased sweating, loss of appetite, nausea, sore throat, tiredness, trouble sleeping, vomiting, or weakness.

Duloxetine is SNRI antidepressant. It works by increasing the amounts of serotonin and norepinephrine, natural substances in the brain that help maintain mental balance and stop the movement of pain signals in the brain.

NORTRIPTYLINE: AVENTYL, PAMELOR

Side effects that may occur while taking this medicine include dry mouth, drowsiness, dizziness, headache, nausea, weakness, diarrhea, excess sweating, heartburn, unpleasant taste, weight gain, or an increased appetite especially for sweets.

This medicine is a tricyclic antidepressant used to treat depression. It may also be used to treat chronic pain.

VENLAFAXINE: EFFEXOR

Side effects that may occur while taking this medicine include anxiety, blurred vision, changes in taste, constipation, decreased sexual desire or ability, dizziness, drowsiness, dry mouth, flushing, headache, increased sweating, loss of appetite, nausea, nervousness, stomach upset, trouble sleeping, vomiting, weakness, weight loss, or yawning.

Venlafaxine is SNRI antidepressant used in the treatment of depression, anxiety, and panic attacks. It works by restoring the balance of natural substances in the brain. Venlafaxine may improve your mood, feelings of well-being, and energy level and decrease nervousness and the number of panic attacks you may have.

AMITRIPTYLINE: ELAVIL, ENDEP, VANATRIP

Side effects that may occur include Nausea vomiting drowsiness, weakness or tiredness, nightmares, headaches, dry mouth, constipation, difficulty urinating, blurred vision, pain, burning or tingling in hands or feet, change in sex drive, excessive sweating, changes in appetite or weight, confusion, unsteadiness,

Amitriptyline is tricyclic antidepressants. It works by increasing the amounts of certain natural substances in the brain that are needed to maintain mental balance. Amitriptyline is also used to treat eating disorders, post-herpetic neuralgia, and to prevent migraine headaches.

There are several anticonvulsant medications that are found very helpful in preventing or reducing migraines and headaches.

DIVALPROEX SODIUM: DEPAKOTE

Side effects that may occur while taking this medicine include change in appetite, constipation, diarrhea, headache, nausea, vomiting, indigestion, stomach cramps or pain, drowsiness, dizziness, trouble sleeping, weight change, weakness, or hair loss.

This medication is used to treat seizure disorders, certain psychiatric conditions and to prevent migraine headaches. It works by restoring the balance of certain natural substances (neurotransmitters) in the brain.

TOPIRAMATE: TOPAMAX, TOPIRAGEN

Side effects that may occur while taking this medicine include constipation, decreased sweating, diarrhea, drowsiness, dry mouth, flu-like symptoms, loss of appetite, nausea, nervousness, numbness and tingling, runny nose, sore throat, stomach pain or upset, taste changes, tiredness, trouble sleeping, or weight loss.

This medicine is an anticonvulsant used alone or with other medicines to control certain types of seizures. It may be also used to prevent migraine headaches.

GABAPENTIN: NEURONTIN, FANATREX, GABARONE, GRALISE, HORIZANT

Side effects that may occur while taking this medication include clumsiness, diarrhea, tiredness, drowsiness, dizziness, nausea, dry mouth, constipation, vomiting, weight gain, or an upset stomach.

Gabapentin was originally developed for the treatment of epilepsy, and currently is also used to relieve neuropathic pain.

Beta blocker drugs are usually prescribed to help control or maintain blood pressure, chest pain. Beta blockers have been found helpful in the prevention of migraines and headaches. Here are a few of the commonly prescribed beta blocker medications used for migraine prevention.

NADOLOL CORGARD

Side effects may include dizziness or lightheadedness, excessive tiredness.

Nadolol works by relaxing blood vessels and slowing heart rate to improve blood flow and decrease blood pressure. Nadolol is also used sometimes to prevent migraine headaches.

PROPRANOLOL: INDERAL, PRONOL, INNOPRAN

Side effects that may occur while taking this medicine include constipation; diarrhea; dizziness; drowsiness; fatigue; lightheadedness; nausea; stomach upset or cramping; trouble sleeping; vomiting; or weakness.

Propanolol is used to treat high blood pressure and chest pain. It is also used after a heart attack and also used to prevent migraine headaches. It works by relaxing blood vessels and slowing heart rate to improve blood flow and decrease blood pressure.

TIMOLOL MALEATE: BLOCADREN

Side effects that may go away during treatment include mild drowsiness; lightheadedness or dizziness; or unusual tiredness or weakness.

Timolol is used to treat high blood pressure and to improve survival after a heart attack. It is also is used to prevent migraine headaches. It works by relaxing blood vessels and slowing heart rate to improve blood flow and decrease blood pressure.

THERAPIES

There are numerous treatments and therapies for migraine and headache sufferers and many more that are still being discovered. Many neurologists go to a variety of headache conferences and seminars to learn more about the vast improvements and new research for migraines and headaches.

Acupuncture is an alternative medicine originated in ancient China over 3,000 years ago. Acupuncture is a series of thin, solid needles that are inserted into acupuncture points in the skin. Stimulating these points can correct imbalances and thought to aid the body's natural healing abilities.

Acupuncture is a concept of Traditional Chinese Medicine. The theory is that bodily functions are regulated by the flow of an energy-like entity called qi, pronounced chee. Qi is the flow of energy or a life-force. The translation of Qi means breath, air or gas.

Acupuncture has been found helpful for migraines and other issues involving pain with and without medications.

Biofeedback is techniques you learn in order to control your pain. Biofeedback is a type of pain management therapy. When you begin learning biofeedback techniques, you learn how to control functions your body does normally. This involves reducing the effects of pain and stress on your body by learning how your body reacts to pain and stress. While training, you use machines to monitor your tension and teach you how to control physical processes that are stress related. Certain exercises such as self-hypnosis and thermal biofeedback are taught to help maintain and prevent migraines naturally. It takes about ten to twenty lessons to learn these techniques effectively. Your doctor can refer you if this is something you are interested in trying.

There is a lot of information regarding biofeedback at http://en.wikipedia.org/wiki/Biofeedback or you can discuss it with doctor.

Botox (onabotulinum toxin type A) is a protein produced by bacterium clostridium botulinum. This is the most powerful neurotoxin found to date. Botox is a prescription medication that is injected into muscles and is FDA approved for migraine prevention in adults with chronic migraines.

In the mid-1990s there were numerous people who received botulinum toxin for other reasons who reported improvements in headaches. Clinical trials of botulinum toxin were performed on people who suffered from various headache types. There were no differences found in the headaches for tension type, episodic migraine, and undifferentiated chronic headache with patients who were given the botulinum toxin verses those given placebo.

In studies of patients with chronic migraine headache, the patients reported decreased pain after treatment with botulinum toxin. It is thought that muscle tension may trigger or aggravate migraine headache and botulinum toxin reduces the headache pain by decreasing the muscle tension.

Your body has a chemical known as acetylcholine which is a neurotransmitter in your peripheral and central nervous systems. Acetylcholine sends signals for muscles to contract. Botulinum toxin binds the nerve endings, blocking the release of acetylcholine. Basically botulinum toxin blocks the message sent for your muscles to contract.

Botox is a treatment given in three month intervals. You are given a series of intramuscular injections in specific "trigger point" areas of your head, face, and the base of skull. Other injections sites are possible as well depending on where your pain is. Aside from the places I just mentions, I also receive injections in my trapezoids' and upper back near my shoulder blades since I also experience pain and tension there as well. Personally speaking I have had good results since beginning Botox treatments. It may not work for everyone and it does require you to be consistent with your treatments. I used to be able to tell when it was almost time for my next Botox treatments. My headaches would tend to increase around two weeks before my next treatment. I have been receiving these injections for several years and they now seem to last until the next treatment. I do still get migraines and headaches however they are definitely less severe and less frequent.

What you need to remember about Botox is that they are injections. The needles used are very small, thin needles. Sometime they tend to hurt a little more than other times. I do not have a fear of needles at all. I have had uncountable tests and treatments throughout the past twenty years; a shot does not faze me in the least. That being said, when you get anywhere between thirty and fifty injections in different spots during one session, you sort of feel like a pin cushion. You get used to it and don't even mind because of the results you get from it. If I have recently had more frequent and painful headaches (for example around hurricane season) I will be tenderer; then the injections will be more painful. During times when my headaches are not that bad and I am less tender the injections don't seem to hurt much at all. Don't allow the thought of multiple injections scare you. It generally takes fifteen minutes for the entire appointment and may be worth it for you to give it a chance. This is not a treatment you can just request. You have to have gone through several types of treatments without good results and your doctor must think you are a candidate as not everyone is.

Occipital Nerve Block is an injection with a steroid around the nerve to temporarily block or inactivate the nerve. The steroid injected reduces the inflammation and swelling of tissue around the occipital nerves. This treatment is generally used for chronic pain. The nerve block usually has an effect on other sensations as well.

Trigger point injections may also be helpful. These involve the injection of an anesthetic agent combined with an anti-inflammatory medication. Some neurologist use Xylocaine mixed with Depomedrol (a steroid) to reduce pain and inflammation in the muscle. These injections are given at trigger points such as the base of the skull and in the temple area. You can get these injections frequently. I get them almost every visit to my neurologist. Often when I get them in the temple area I do have a metallic taste and mild dizziness for a short while after the injections. The first time that happened it scared me. It seems to be a side effect from the injection and does subside.

Steroid treatment is usually used in order to break up a bad bout of migraine or headache. When you have had a severe migraine or several severe migraines for a period of time without relief your doctor may prescribe a "steroid burst" which is when you take a prescription oral steroid at a large dose. For example, you may be prescribed to take prednisolone. It will most likely be a 7-day burst meaning for example you will start by taking four pills at a moderate dose on the first and second day, the third and fourth day you will take three doses, fifth day you take two doses and take one dose on the final two days. This is supposed to break up the migraine.

Oral prednisolone is a corticosteroid and an anti-inflammatory drug. There are side effects for steroids in general such as weight gain. While on the burst you will notice rather quickly, possibly by the very first dose, that you are bloating. The rings on your fingers may become uncomfortable and tight. You may also experience that you are hungry more frequently than usual. You may experience mood swings or feelings of agitation. I tend to have an adverse reaction when I take oral steroids. I am fine on the first day however I begin having a bloody nose several times a day. It is not bad, but bad enough. So I stay away from oral steroids if possible. They have been known to help in many situations.

Occipital Nerve stimulation is a surgical procedure where a small device is implanted at the base of the skull. This is a fairly new procedure for headache purposes. The implanted device gives a small electrical charge to the occipital nerve to prevent migraines and headaches for people who have not responded to medications.

Reference & Resources
**Helpful websites and Books

National Headache Foundation
www.headaches.org

Migraine Awareness group (MAGNUM)
www.migraines.org

American Migraine Foundation
www.americanheadachefoundation.org

The Migraine Trust
www.migrainetrust.org

National Center for Biotechnology Information, U.S. National Library of Medicine
www.ncbi.nlm.nih.gov

Mountain Rose Herbs
www.mountainroseherbs.com

Med Central
www.medcentral.org

www.relieve-migraine-headaches.com

www.livingstrong.com

www.patientslikeme.com

www.walgreens.com

www.uhc.com

www.weather.com

The Pill Book Editor-in-chief, Harold M. Silverman

Herbal Remedies by Andrew Chevallier

P

Peppermint, 62

Q

Qi, 89

R

Rosemary, 63

S

SNRI, 82, 83, 84
Stadol, 80
Status Migraine, 8
Steroid, 93

Symptoms, 40

T

Tension headache, 12
Tramadol, 80
Triggers, 55
Triptans, 67

V

Venlafaxine, 84
Vicodin, 26

X

Xylocaine, 93